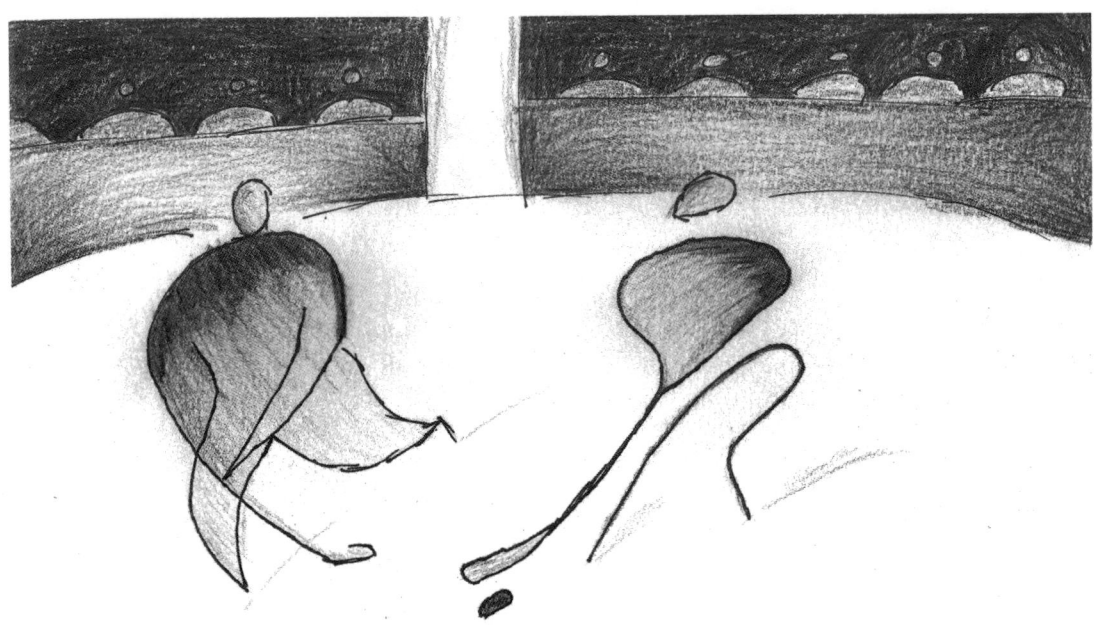

Jonathan Linton odibaajimowin imaa Mistaasiniing
The Story of Jonathan Linton of Mistissini

Told by Jonathan Linton
Written by Ruth DyckFehderau
Translated into Ojibwe by Patricia M. Ningewance

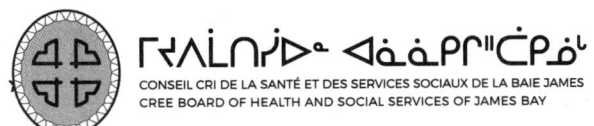

ᒥᓯᐱᓂᑭᐦᐃᐧᐃᒃ ᐊᑖᓇᐱᒋᐦᑕᐹᓇ
CONSEIL CRI DE LA SANTÉ ET DES SERVICES SOCIAUX DE LA BAIE JAMES
CREE BOARD OF HEALTH AND SOCIAL SERVICES OF JAMES BAY

Funding for this publication was provided in part by Health Canada. The opinions expressed in this publication are those of the storyteller and do not necessarily reflect the official views of Health Canada or of the Cree Board of Health and Social Services of James Bay.

First printing, 2020. Printed and bound in Canada by Houghton Boston Printers, Saskatoon, Saskatchewan. Distributed by Wilfrid Laurier University Press / wlupress.wlu.ca

Set in Verdana font, chosen for its readability. Printed on paper that is Forest Stewardship Council-certified with post-consumer recycled fibres, and that is acid- and chlorine-free.

Cover design by Nicole Ritzer, based on an original design by Cameron Mosimann. Photograph of Mistissini burnt forest (reversed) taken by David DyckFehderau. Title page illustration by Semera Coon of Mikw Chiyâm Arts Concentration Program, Voyageur Memorial High School, Mistissini, QC.

Published by Cree Board of Health and Social Services of James Bay
Contact: Paul Linton, 168 Main St, Mistissini, QC, Canada, G0W 1C0 / (418) 923-3355
creehealth.org / sweetbloods.org

Library and Archives Canada Cataloguing in Publication

Title: Jonathan Linton odibaajimowin imaa Mistaasiniing = The story of Jonathan Linton of Mistissini / written, Ruth DyckFehderau o-gii-ozhibii'aan ; told, Jonathan Linton ; translated into Ojibwe, Patricia M. Ningewance.

Other titles: Story of Jonathan Linton of Mistissini

Names: DyckFehderau, Ruth, author. | Container of (work): DyckFehderau, Ruth. Story of Jonathan Linton of Mistissini. | Container of (expression): DyckFehderau, Ruth. Story of Jonathan Linton of Mistissini. Ojibwa. | Cree Board of Health and Social Services of James Bay, publisher.

Description: "A Story from The Sweet Bloods of Eeyou Istchee: Stories of Diabetes and the James Bay Cree." | Text in Ojibwa and English.

Identifiers: Canadiana 2020021831X | ISBN 9780973054279 (softcover)

Subjects: LCSH: Linton, Jonathan (Of Mistissini)—Health. | LCSH: Diabetics—Cree Nation of Mistissini—Biography. | LCGFT: Biographies.

Classification: LCC RC660 .D93 2020 | DDC 362.1964/620092—dc23

Odaabaaning onji-gabaa Jonathan. Imaa bakekana awi-niibawi ezhiishiigid imaa gooning edagwaagig. Gaa-ishkwaa-zhigid apan miinawaa boozi, odeden dash miinawaa maajiibizowan. Onjida bejibizowag e-nanaandone'amowaad awensiwan ji-nametoonid bakekana. Maagizhaa gaag maagizhaa gaye bine. Ambegish naa moonz. Gaamashi moonzoon obaashkizwaasiin Jonathan. Odebibidoon onibiim e-minikwed nibi. Wiinge naa bengwanaamo. Zhebaa o-gii-nisaawaa niizhin nika', odaanaang imaa abiwag. Aazha miinawaa maajiibizowag nishikaach.

Aazha miinawaa wii-zhigi Jonathan. Aazha miinawaa gibichiiwan odeden.

Ozazaamakamig.

Aazha nishwaaching zhigi noongom ango-diba'igan gaa-izhisenig. Ozazaamakamig. Gaawn editawe awiya daa-apiichi-niibiwa-zhigisii? Wiinge gaye bengwanaamo. Odaana-gagwe-mikwendaan wegonen wenji-ayaad imaa, e-gii'osed. Aazha moozhag gii'ose. O-gii-baashkizwaabaniin binen nitam gii-ngodwaaso-bibooned. Wiinge dash maanamanji'o aana-gagwe-gii'osed.

Bengodoone. Bizhishig zhiishiigi. Ngoji o-gii-agindaanaaban ini ikidowinan. Oooh, ziizibaakwadwaapinewin dazhinjigaadeban

Jonathan stepped out of the truck, sidled up to a bush, unzipped his jeans, and peed into the October snow. He zipped up, climbed back into the truck, and his dad slid it into gear again. They drove slowly, looking out carefully for tracks or disturbed foliage, any hint that a porcupine or partridge had passed by. Moose would be nice. Jonathan still hadn't shot a moose. He twisted the cap off his water bottle and sucked back a mouthful. Strange how dry his mouth was. This morning's kill, a pair of geese, sat in the back of the truck. They inched forward again.

Except – Jonathan had to pee. Again. His dad stopped the truck.

This was ridiculous.

He'd peed *eight* times in the last hour. How could one human body even make that much pee? What was the point in doing up his fly if he was just gonna have to pee again? And his mouth. He could write a letter on his tongue, it was so dry. Focus, he told himself. Jonathan had done quite a bit of hunting. Shot his first partridge when he was six. Now, he knew, was the time to concentrate – but he felt *awful*.

Dry mouth. Frequent urination. He'd seen those words somewhere on a list. No, on a poster about – diabetes? Jonathan was

mazina'iiginong. Gaawiin wiin.
Onzaam wiin oshkaadizi gaye bizhishig
babaa-gii'ose. Gaawiin wiin. Midaashi-
naano-biboone Jonathan, gikino'amaagozi
gaye ishpi-gikino'amaadiiwigamigong
imaa Mistaasinii Makwa
zhooshkwaada'ewininiwag izhi-wiijitwaa.
Gaawiin wiin daa-ziizibaakwadwaapinesii.

Gaawiin na tagiin?

Ngojigo nisogon e-izhisenig namadabi
Jonathan adoopowining endaad.
Odayaan zhaabonigan gaye gegoonan
gaa-biindegin imaa makakoonsing
gaa-gii-ondinang mashkikiiwigamigong
ji-gagwe-gikendang aaniin
ezhinaagwaninig omiskwiim, aaniin
minik ziizibaakwad eyaamaganinig.
Jiita'odizo. Ozhizhoonaan omiskwiim
imaa mazina'iiginoonsing. Ogikendaan
giishpin ngojigo naanan izhisenig,
onizhishinini. Giishpin dash wiin
6 biinish 7 izhisenig, gaawiin aapiji
onizhishinzinoon. Giishpin dash
wiin awashime 7 izhisenig, amii
eziizibaakwadwaapined.

Oganawaabandaan iweni gaa-
ozhibii'igaadenig ezhisenig omiskwiim.
32.3 izhibii'igaadeni. Ozazaamakamig.
Gaawn editawe. Giishpin awashime
30 izhisenig aakoziiwigamigong
zhemaak daa-izhiwinaa. Maagizhaa
daa-nepidingwaamise. Aazha miinawaa
odoodaapinaan omiskwiim. 32.1 noongom

young and fit and healthy. A 15-year-old
hunter and high school student and
enforcer on the Mistissini Bears hockey
team. It couldn't be diabetes.

Could it?

A few days later, Jonathan sat at the
kitchen table and read the instructions on
a diabetes test kit. He inserted a test strip
into the glucometer device, unwrapped
the lancet in the kit, and pricked his
finger. He carefully smeared some blood
onto the test strip. A blood sugar level
below 6 was normal, he knew, between
6 and 7 was pre-diabetes, a warning sign
that diabetes was just around the corner,
and anything over 7 was diabetes.

He looked at the glucometer. It said his
blood sugar level was 32.2. That couldn't
be right. A reading of over 30 meant he
had to be hospitalized immediately because
he could slip into a coma. He took the test
again. 32.1. And again and again and again.
All the numbers were about the same. No
question, Jonathan had diabetes.

izhiseni. Miinawaa gii-izhichige. Miinawaa dash. Amii go bizhishig iwe minik gaa-inaagoshkaanig iwe gaa-waabandang. Ziizibaakwadwaapine ngwana Jonathan.

Bazigwii. Apane gii-izhaa wedi mashkikiiwigamigong. Ziizibaakwadwaapine mashkiki zhemaak o-gii-miinaawaan. Ango-diba'igan e-izhisenig nawach babenag inamanji'o.

He got up from his chair, went to the clinic, where they injected him with insulin. An hour later, he felt better.

Aaniin dash ge-izhichiged. Giishpin iwe apiichi-ishpaakoshkaanig omiskwiim Shibogamaang aakoziiwigamigong gosha daa-ayaa ji-naagaji'igopan mashkikiiwininiwa' gaye mashkikiiwikwe'. Omaamaan CHR inanokiiwan, imaa ishkoniganing ji-wiiji'aad anishinaabe' mino-ayaawining inake inanokii. O-daa-wiindamaagoon aakoziiwigamigong ji-izhaad. Aazha dash gii-giizhaakonigeban Montreal e-wii-izhi-wiijiiwaad owiijiiwaagana' ji-ando-ganawaabamaawaad Montreal Alouettes gaa-izhinikaazowaad odaminowaad. Aazha gii-inaakonigeban ji-wiidoopamaawaad bezhig ini gaa-odaminonid imaa gaye ji-wiiji-mazinaateshimind imaa. Gichi-gegoon iwe. Gaawiin wii-banizisii.

But now he had a problem: his blood sugar levels meant that he should be in the Chibougamau hospital where the doctors and nurses could watch him. His mother was a Community Health Representative (CHR), and she would make him go, he was sure – and that would ruin his weekend plans. He and some friends from football camp were going to Montréal to watch the Montréal Alouettes game and then all meet with them. Jonathan would have supper with the quarterback and be in a commercial with him. It was a big deal and he didn't want to miss it.

O-gii-maajii-zhaagoozomaan omaamaan. Nin-ga-maajiidoonan zhaaboniganan gaye iwe ziizibaakwadwaapine-mashkiki odinaan. Nin-ga-jiita'odiz gwayak. Gi-ga-ozhibii'amawin bizhishig, odinaan.

Methodically, purposefully, he began to persuade his mom to let him go on the trip. He could take needles and insulin, he reasoned. He would follow the injection rules perfectly. He would text

3

Gego gegoon inendangen odinaan. Giishpin gegoon izhiseg baatiinadanoon aakoziiwigamigoon imaa Montreal. Amii gaa-izhi-zhaagoozomaad omaamaan.

Bakaan onaagajitoon. Gaawiin awiyan o-wii-wiindamawaasiin e-ziizibaakwadwaapined. O-gii-gaadoon iwe ni mashkiki omashkimoding, nitam azhiganing e-gii-gashkiiginang miinawaa dash obiitawidaasaaning e-gii-izhi-gashkiiginang. Gaawiin awiya o-daa-waabandanziin. Debwe o-gii-ozhibii'amawaan omaamaan bizhishig. Giishpin gaaskizigan amwag, da-ishpaagoshkaana nimiskwiim? Eya, izhibii'igewan omaamaan. Giishpin dash wiin zhaashaagomikiweyaan? Gaawiin ikidowan. Gaawiin awiyan o-gii-wiindamawaasiin. Owiijiiwaagana', gaye awe gaa-ogimaakandan gii-izhaawaad wedi, gaye awe gaa-odaminod Alouettes. Gaawiin gaye aapiji o-gii-odaapinanziin iweni mashkiki. Wiininong daa-izhisemagan iwe mashkiki, inendam. Gaawiin dash ni-wiininosii. Ni-mashkawewagiz, inendam. Gaawiin dash deminik mashkiki odoodaapinanziin onzaam agaji ji-waabamind jiita'odizod.

Gii-minose iwe gii-izhaawaad imaa gii-ando-waabandamowaad iwe odaminowin. Gaawiin gii-aakozisii Jonathan. Gii-dagoshing endaad

her throughout the weekend and keep her updated. She didn't need to be afraid for him, he'd be careful, he'd be okay. Besides, if anything went wrong, Montréal had hospitals. In the end, she came around.

He still had another problem, though: he needed to keep the diabetes secret. He packed the insulin carefully, tucking it first inside a sock and then rolling the socks into underwear, stuffing it all way down in his bag, where no one would see it. All weekend long, he faithfully texted his mom for advice. Did toast affect blood sugar? (Yes) Did chewing gum affect blood sugar? (No) But he told no one about the diabetes, not his friends, not the trip organizers, and certainly not the Alouettes quarterback. And he didn't take the insulin nearly as often as he should have. *It's hard to inject*, he said to himself. *Insulin has to go into fat. I'm an athlete. Lots of muscle, not a lot of fat.* But in truth, he wasn't taking enough insulin because he didn't want to be seen with insulin.

The football trip was fine and Jonathan didn't get sick, but when he came home, he headed straight for the bedroom and flipped on the TV. And stayed there for zhemaak gaa-izhi-nibaad gii-izhaa. Gaa-mazinaatesenig o-gii-ganawaabandaan. Amii imaa gaa-ayaad. Gaawiin gii-ando-gikino'amaagozisii. Gaawiin gaye gii-izhaasii zhooshkwaada'ewigamigong ji-ando-gagwejiid. Gaawiin gaye ziizibaakwadwaapine-mashkikiiwininiwan o-gii-waabamaasiin.

Biinish ani-maanzhimaagwanini gaa-izhi-nibaad. Gaawiin aaniish onji-zaaga'anzii imaa.

Niizho-dwaate gii-izhisenig odeden oganoonigoon. "Inashke. Gaawiin da-maajaamagazinoon giziizibaakwadwaapinewin michi-ganawaabandaman gaa-mazinaateseg. Gikino'amaadiiwigamigong izhaan. Giiyaabi gi-daa-mino-bimaadiz aanawi aakoziyin. Giizhitooyin gi-gikino'amaagoziwin gi-ga-debinaan anokiiwin. Gego bagijiiken onzaam e-ayaayin iwe inaapinewin."

E-ani-waabaninig gii-izhaa gikino'amaadiiwigamigong Jonathan. Gikino'amaage-ogimaan ogagwejimigoon aandi gaa-ayaad. "Mashkikiiwigamigong nin-gii-izhaa. Amii dash gaa-izhi-abiyaan endaayaan," odinaan. Gaawiin o-giiwiindamawaasiin e-ziizibaakwadwaapined.

O-gii-ando-waabamaan dash ziizibaakwadwaapine-mashkikiiwikwen

days. He didn't go to school. He didn't go to his hockey practices. He didn't go to his hockey games. He didn't see a diabetes specialist.

After a week, his bedroom began to smell a bit ripe.

After two weeks, his dad said, "Look. Television doesn't actually make diabetes go away. Go to school. You can still do everything you did before, you can still be whatever you want to be, unless you don't finish high school. Diabetes isn't the end of the world."

The next day, Jonathan was back in school and playing hockey again. The school principal asked where he'd been. "I went to the clinic and then I stayed home," he said, and looked away. No way was he saying *anything* about diabetes.

He went to a diabetes specialist that week too. She said that some people can

5

naanaage iwe edwaateg. Aaninda awiyag obwaawitoonaawaa iwe ziizibaakwadwaapinewin giishpin aanjitoowaad gaa-inanjigewaad, gaye gagwejiiwaad bizhishig. Giin dash wiin gi-daa-amwaag mashkikiwag gemaa ji-jiita'odizoyin ji-odaapinaman iwe insulin gaa-izhinikaadeg ziizibaakwadwaapine-mashkiki. Giiyaw onji-ozhi'oomagan iwe insulin gaa-izhinikaadeg. Imaa gibiskwading izhi-ozhi'oomagan. Gii-ziizibaakwadwaapineyin dash gaawiin imaa deminik ozhi'oomagazinoon. Amii ezhi-booni-anokiimagak gi-biskwad. Amii dash ezhi-jiita'odizod awe gaa-inaapined.

"Ganage nawach daa-minose giishpin zhemaak maajii-odaapinamaan iwe insulin, ji-jiita'odizoyaan? Nawach nin-daa-mino-doodaan nimbiskwad," odinaan Jonathan.

"Eya," ikido mashkikiiwikwe. "Gi-gikendaan na dash aaniin dasing ge-jiita'odizo'amban?"

Wiinge onagajitoon gii-zhooshkwaada'ed Jonathan, gii-odaminowaad mikomiing. Wiin ako niigaan gaa-babaamaada'ed e-bakiteweba'ang iweni gaa-babaamiweba'amowaad mikomiing. Gaawiin gegoon ogotanziin. Gaawiin o-da-gotanziinan zhaaboniganan. Gaawiin eta onandawenimaasii' godag awiya' ji-waabandaminid.

eventually control diabetes by changing their diet and increasing exercise, but for now Jonathan would have to take either pills or insulin, and most people started with pills. His body needed more insulin, insulin is made in the pancreas, and pills would make the pancreas work harder. Eventually it would burn out, she said, and pancreas burnout is when people usually start injecting insulin with needles.

"Wouldn't it make more sense," Jonathan asked, "if I skipped pills and just injected insulin? I'd be giving my pancreas a break."

"Yes," she said, "but do you know how many needles that will be?"

Jonathan was used to flying pucks, body checks, concussions, broken limbs, and bruises. He was the enforcer on his hockey team, the goon. His job was to do the hitting on the ice, and even to try to aggravate players on the other team and make them screw up. A bunch of little needles every day were not a big deal. As long as no one saw them.

Gwayak gii-maajii-inanjige, gaawiin aapiji bakwezhiganan, opiniin gaye waabi-manoominan, iwe dinookaan miijim. Gaawiin gaye o-gii-miijisiin adaawewigamigong gaa-adaawaadeg abinoojiiyag gaa-minopidamowaad. O-gii-odaapinaan omashkikiim dasing gii-wiisinid miinawaa jibwaa-gawishimod. Nawach gaye bizhishig gii-gagwejii. Ngojigo niso-giizis gii-izhisenig aabita eta iwe insulin o-gii-aabajitoon. Biinish ango-giizis gii-izhisenig, aabita miinawaa minik insulin gii-inaa ji-aabajitood. Biinish gaawiin memwaach o-gii-aabajitoosiin iweni mashkiki. Aapiji o-gii-gashkitoon ji-ani-mino-ayaad. Giiyaabi dash gaawiin awiya bakaan o-gii-wiindamawaasiin ezhiiyaad. Oniigi'igoo' eta.

Gaawiin awiya bakaan o-daa-gikendanziin, inendam. Giishpin awiya gikendang gikino'amaadiiwigamigong nin-ga-onji-miikinzomigoo gemaa nin-ga-miigaanigoo. Giishpin awiya bangii bakaan izhiiyaad, amii ezhi-miikinzomaawaad. Daabishkoo awe ikwezens bezhig. Gii-maajii-mazinibii'odizod owadengong, bishigwaachikwe o-gii-izhinikaanaawaan. Aazha gaye nin-gii-miigaanig bezhig gichi-gwiiwizens onzaam aabita e-wemitigoozhiiwiyaan. Giishpin gikendamowaad eziizibaakwadwaapineyaan nin-ga-miigaanigoo, inendam.

Jonathan began to eat more carefully – fewer carbohydrates, less junk food, less frequent snacking – and took his insulin religiously, one shot every time he ate and another before bed. He worked out even more than he had before. After a few months, he needed about half as much insulin and another month later, half of that. Soon he wasn't using insulin or any diabetes medication at all. He had made important progress: he had brought severe diabetes under control. But he still didn't tell anyone that he had the disease.

It has to be secret, he said to himself as he bench-pressed the barbell. *It's dangerous to tell people,* he thought, hoisting his chin over the chin-up bar. Anybody at school who was a little bit different was bullied regularly. Like that girl who got harassed and called a slut just because she wore a bit of eye makeup. The toughest guy in school was already beating Jonathan up for being half-Cree, half-white. *If they find out I'm diabetic too, I'll never make it home,* he thought, straining against the plates on the leg machine.

Aabiding dash gikino'amaadiiwigamigong e-dazhi-giziininjiid wenji-biindiged awe gaa-nitaa-miigaanigod gichi-gwiiwizensan. Obasijiishkaagoon. "Wemichigoozhiwish!" odigoon.

Amii gaa-izhi-nanaakwiid Jonathan. Onishki'igoon bizhishig egagwaadagi'igod. Bizhishig gii-gagwejiid gii-onji-mashkawizii. Ezhi-bakitewaad oskatigoning. Apane gaa-gawised awe godag. Gii-babimishin ajina imaa. Gii-bazigwii. Gaawiin miinawaa wiikaa o-gii-babaamenimigosiin. Ngoding dash o-gii-maajitoonaawaa izhichigewin imaa gikino'amaadiiwigamigong ji-booni-gagwaadagi'iwewaad gaa-mindidowaad gikino'amawaaganag. Ani-aanjise noongom omaa, inendam Jonathan. Maagizhaa bizaanigo daa-wiindamaage enaapined.

Aabiding dash o-gii-maajii-wiindamawaan bezhig owiijiiwaaganan e-ayaad iwe inaapinewin. "Hah," eta ikidowan. Amii dash bakaan gaa-izhi-maajii-doodaagod. Gaawiin noongom o-wii-wiijiiwigosiin, daabishkoo egotaajinid ji-aazhoo'aad. Gaawiin iinzan aaninda gegoonan da-aanjisesinoonan inendam. Amii ndawaa eta awiya wiindamawaasiwag ge-izhi-onizhishing inendam.

Gii-midaashi-naano-bibooned makwan o-gii-nisaan. Ngojigo

At school one day, Jonathan stood at the sink in the bathroom. The door swung open and the toughest guy in school walked in and came at Jonathan as he had so many times before. "White boy" he jeered, and kneed him in the stomach.

Jonathan didn't think about how frustrated he was with the tough guy, nor about his diabetes secret, nor about how much stronger all the extra workouts had made him. He just wound up and landed one solid punch to the forehead. The guy buckled and hit the ground. He lay there on his back for a while, then got up and never bothered Jonathan again. Soon after that, the school brought in an anti-bullying program. Things were beginning to change. Jonathan began to think about letting his secret out.

Tentatively, hesitantly, Jonathan mentioned to one of his friends that he had diabetes. "Huh," his friend said – and began avoiding him, as if he had something contagious instead of diabetes. Some things, like being treated badly in high school if you were different, would probably never change. For Jonathan, secrecy was still the way to go.

The year Jonathan turned 16, he killed a bear. 24 feet away, 7 mm with a scope.

nishtana-shi-niiwi-mizid gii-onjigaabawi gii-baashkizwaad 7 mm dinookaan baashkizigan e-gii-aabajitood. Ganawaabam makwa ji-waabamig jibwaa-baashkizwad gii-inaa iinzan. Giiyaabi gaawiin awiyan miinawaa o-gii-wiindamawaasiin gaa-inaapined.

Gii-midaashi-niizhwaaso-bibooned, Junior AAA gaa-izhinikaadeg gaa-bimaada'ewaad o-gii-andawenimigoo' ji-niigaanaada'ed. Gaawiin dash gii-minosesinoon. Baamaa miinawaa nin-ga-gojitoon gii-inendam. O-gii-minwendaan dash wiin igo e-gii-gagwejimind. Aazha miinawaa o-gii-maajii-odaapinaan iwe insulin. Giiyaabi gaawiin gii-wiindamaagesii.

Ngojigo iwe apii, Cree Board of Health, gaa-gikendamowaad eziizibaakwadwaapinenid Jonathan o-gii-gagwejimigoo' ji-dibaadodang iwe ziizibaakwadwaapinewin ji-gikendamowaad CHR gaa-inanokiiwaad. Ahaaw gii-ikido. Meshkwach dash gaawiin awiya da-wiindamaagesii aweneniwid, ji-dibaajimind. Eya, gii-ikidowa'. Apii gii-gaagiigidod o-gii-dazhindaan aaniin enendang gii-inaapined iwe, gaye e-wiindamaaged wegonen igo aazha gaa-gikendang.

Ngojigo niiwing iwe gii-izhichiged, gii-izhaa imaa gaa-izhi-gagwejiid gii-zhooshkwaada'ed. E-ani-giiwed,

Like the elders taught, he was careful to make full eye contact with the bear before shooting. The diabetes was still a secret.

The year Jonathan turned 17, a Junior AAA hockey team wanted him to be their enforcer. It didn't work out, and he could try again next year, but it was nice to be asked. That year, he had to start taking insulin again too. And the diabetes was still a secret.

Around that time, the Cree Board of Health (which had record of his diabetes) asked Jonathan to give some presentations about his diabetes to Community Health Representatives and nurses. He agreed, but only if no one outside the room would find out. In every presentation, to every roomful of healthcare workers, he described his experiences and gave all the insight and information that he could – but asked that each person in the room keep his condition confidential. Secrecy was so much work.

After the fourth presentation, he went to hockey practice. A few hours later, on the way home, he dropped his heavy o-gii-bagijiwebinaan omashkimod imaa miikanaang. Ogijibidoon ogiigidowin amii dash gaa-izhi-ozhibii'ang imaa Facebook e-ziizibaakwadwaapined.

Amii sa gakina awiya ji-gikendang. Amii gii-wiindamaaged.

Igi gaa-wiijiiwaad gii-bimaada'ed, gaawiin gegoon o-gii-inendanziinaawaa. Deminik nagadaada'ed, amii deminik ezhi-onizhishing gii-inendamoog. Odikwezensiman gaye aazha o-gii-gikendaan, gaawiin gewiin gegoon o-gii-inendanziin. O-mino-doodaagoon ogwiiwizensiman, gaawiin o-daa-onji-majenimaasiin iwe e-inaapinenid.

Iya'aan eta bezhig gikino'amaagewininiwan bezhigwan gaa-inaapinenid o-gii-onji'igoon ji-zhooshkwaada'esig. "Gaawiin gi-daa-zhooshkwaada'esiimin giinawind iwe gaa-inaapineying," o-gii-igoon. "Onzaam zanagan. Maagizhaa gi-daa-wiisagaapinanigoo."

Aapiji wii-baapi'aan ini gaa-ikidonid. Niizho-biboon gaawiin memwaach o-gii-odaapinanziin iweni insulin mashkiki onzaam bizhishig e-gii-zhooshkwaada'ed enigok e-odaminod mikomiing. Amii iwe gii-gichi-zhooshkwaada'ed gii-babaamibani'od mikomiing gaa-gii-onji-mino-ayaad. Gaawiin nin-ga-bizindawaasii awe inini inendam Jonathan. Gewiin

equipment bag on the sidewalk, pulled out his cellphone, and posted on Facebook that he, Jonathan Linton, had diabetes.

There was no going back. Now, everyone knew.

His hockey team, it turned out, didn't actually care. If he was still the best enforcer around, if he still struck fear into the opposing team, it didn't matter. His girlfriend, who had known for a while but kept the secret, also didn't care. If he treated her well, what did it matter?

What was more surprising was the response of a high school teacher who himself had diabetes: "You know," the teacher said one day, "We diabetics shouldn't play hockey. It's too rough."

It was all Jonathan could do not to laugh. He didn't mean to be rude but he had gone for two years without medication or insulin because of his exercise regime. The exercise had brought his blood sugar levels down. At first, Jonathan thought, *Well, I can't really bother with this guy too much anymore*. The *Aha*! moment came a little later. If a high odayaan iwe inaapinewin, aapiji gaye gikendaaso e-gikino'amaagewininiiwid, giiyaabi dash gaawiin debwe onisidotanziin aaniin ezhiiyaamagak iwe inaapinewin. Ndawaach nin-daa-gii-babaa-dazhindaan ezhi-gikendamaan iwe inaapinewin, inendam.

Amii dash noongom ezhichiged Jonathan CHR e-inanokiid. Ominwendaan odanokiiwin. Naagaji'idizo iwe gewiin gii-ayaad ziizibaakwadwaapinewin. Niibiwa awiya' o-babaa-ganoonaa' e-wiiji'aad. Owendendaan noongom e-dazhindang ziizibaakwadwaapinewin. Odaanaang gaa-dwaateg CBC bizinjiganing gii-noondaagozi e-dazhindang iweni. Obimigiizhitoon gaye ogikino'amaagoowin endaad e-onji-gikino'amaagozid. Heather Hughboy izhinikaazowan odikwezensiman, wii-oniijaanisiwan. Ozhiitaa e-wii-odedemaawid. Giiyaabi gaye wii-zhooshkwaada'e. Gaye wii-gii'ose. Aazha gaagwan o-gii-nisaan, makwan, amikwan, adikwan niibiwa giiyaabi. Gaawiin dash eta mashi moonzoon onisaasiin.

school teacher, an educated educator with plenty of experience in diabetes, believed something so completely false about the disease, it was time to start talking about diabetes.

Nowadays, Jonathan works as a CHR for the Cree Board of Health. He loves the work. It reminds him to take care of his own health, and he's able to meet people and help out them out. He talks about diabetes easily now, and to anyone who wants to hear about it. Just last week, he gave an interview in Cree on CBC radio. He's finishing up high school on the side through homeschooling. His girlfriend, Heather Hughboy, is pregnant; he's getting ready to be a dad and to play more hockey. And to hunt. He's killed porcupine, bear, beaver, caribou, and more – but still no moose.